Keto Chaffle Recipes Cookbook for Beginners

Simple, Easy and Irresistible Low Carb and Gluten Free Ketogenic Waffle Recipes to Lose Weight

Jennifer Hudson

Table of Content

6

RECIPES

Beginners

Chocolate Melt Chaffles

Preparation Time: 15 minutes

Cooking Time: 36 minutes

Servings: 4

Ingredients

For the chaffles:

- 2 eggs, beaten
- ¼ cup finely grated Gruyere cheese
- 2 tbsp heavy cream
- 1 tbsp coconut flour
- 2 tbsp cream cheese, softened
- 3 tbsp unsweetened cocoa powder
- 2 tsp vanilla extract
- A pinch of salt

For the chocolate sauce:

- 1/3 cup + 1 tbsp heavy cream
- 1 ½ oz unsweetened baking chocolate, chopped
- 1 ½ tsp sugar-free maple syrup
- 1 ½ tsp vanilla extract

Directions:

For the chaffles:

1. Preheat the waffle iron.
2. In a medium bowl, mix all the ingredients for the chaffles.
3. Open the iron and add a quarter of the mixture. Close and cook until crispy, 7 minutes.
4. Transfer the chaffle to a plate and make 3 more with the remaining batter.

For the chocolate sauce:

1. Pour the heavy cream into saucepan and simmer over low heat, 3 minutes.
2. Turn the heat off and add the chocolate. Allow melting for a few minutes and stir until fully melted, 5 minutes.
3. Mix in the maple syrup and vanilla extract.
4. Assemble the chaffles in layers with the chocolate sauce sandwiched between each layer.
5. Slice and serve immediately.

Nutrition:

Calories 172

Fats 13.57g

Carbs 6.65g

Net Carbs 3.65g

Protein 5.76g

Chaffles with Keto Ice Cream

Preparation Time: 10 minutes

Cooking Time: 14 minutes

Servings: 2

Ingredients:

- 1 egg, beaten
- ½ cup finely grated mozzarella cheese
- ¼ cup almond flour
- 2 tbsp swerve confectioner's sugar
- 1/8 tsp xanthan gum
- Low-carb ice cream (flavor of your choice) for serving

Directions:

1. Preheat the waffle iron.
2. In a medium bowl, mix all the ingredients except the ice cream.
3. Open the iron and add half of the mixture. Close and cook until crispy, 7 minutes.
4. Transfer the chaffle to a plate and make second one with the remaining batter.
5. On each chaffle, add a scoop of low carb ice cream, fold into half-moons and enjoy.

Nutrition:

Calories 89

Net Carbs 1.37g

Fats 6.48g

Protein 5.91g

Carbs 1.67g

Strawberry Shortcake Chaffle Bowls

Preparation Time: 10 minutes

Cooking Time: 28 minutes

Servings: 4

Ingredients:

- 1 egg, beaten
- ½ cup finely grated mozzarella cheese
- 1 tbsp almond flour
- ¼ tsp baking powder
- 2 drops cake batter extract
- 1 cup cream cheese, softened
- 1 cup fresh strawberries, sliced
- 1 tbsp sugar-free maple syrup

Directions:

1. Preheat a waffle bowl maker and grease lightly with cooking spray.
2. Meanwhile, in a medium bowl, whisk all the ingredients except the cream cheese and strawberries.
3. Open the iron, pour in half of the mixture, cover, and cook until crispy, 6 to 7 minutes.
4. Remove the chaffle bowl onto a plate and set aside.
5. Make a second chaffle bowl with the remaining batter.
6. To serve, divide the cream cheese into the chaffle bowls and top with the strawberries.
7. Drizzle the filling with the maple syrup and serve.

Nutrition:

Calories 235

Fats 20.62g

Carbs 5.9g

Net Carbs 5g

Protein 7.51g

Blueberry Chaffles

Preparation Time: 10 minutes

Cooking Time: 28 minutes

Servings: 4

Ingredients:

- 1 egg, beaten
- ½ cup finely grated mozzarella cheese
- 1 tbsp cream cheese, softened
- 1 tbsp sugar-free maple syrup + extra for topping
- ½ cup blueberries
- ¼ tsp vanilla extract

Directions:

1. Preheat the waffle iron.
2. In a medium bowl, mix all the ingredients.
3. Open the iron, lightly grease with cooking spray and pour in a quarter of the mixture.
4. Close the iron and cook until golden brown and crispy, 7 minutes.
5. Remove the chaffle onto a plate and set aside.
6. Make the remaining chaffles with the remaining mixture.
7. Drizzle the chaffles with maple syrup and serve afterward.

<u>Nutrition:</u>

Calories 137

Fats 9.07g

Carbs 4.02g

Net Carbs 3.42g

Protein 9.59g

Chaffles with Raspberry Syrup

Preparation Time: 10 minutes

Cooking Time: 38 minutes

Servings: 4

Ingredients:

For the chaffles:

- 1 egg, beaten
- ½ cup finely shredded cheddar cheese
- 1 tsp almond flour
- 1 tsp sour cream

For the raspberry syrup:

- 1 cup fresh raspberries
- ¼ cup swerve sugar
- ¼ cup water
- 1 tsp vanilla extract

Directions:

For the chaffles:

1. Preheat the waffle iron.
2. Meanwhile, in a medium bowl, mix the egg, cheddar cheese, almond flour, and sour cream.
3. Open the iron, pour in half of the mixture, cover, and cook until crispy, 7 minutes.
4. Remove the chaffle onto a plate and make another with the remaining batter.

For the raspberry syrup:

1. Meanwhile, add the raspberries, swerve sugar, water, and vanilla extract to a medium pot. Set over low heat and cook until the raspberries soften and sugar becomes syrupy. Occasionally stir while mashing the raspberries as you go. Turn the heat off when your desired consistency is achieved and set aside to cool.
2. Drizzle some syrup on the chaffles and enjoy when ready.

Nutrition:

Calories 105

Fats 7.11g

Carbs 4.31g

Net Carbs 2.21g

Protein 5.83g

Chaffle Cannoli

Preparation Time: 15 minutes

Cooking Time: 28 minutes

Servings: 4

Ingredients:

For the chaffles:

- 1 large egg
- 1 egg yolk
- 3 tbsp butter, melted
- 1 tbso swerve confectioner's
- 1 cup finely grated Parmesan cheese
- 2 tbsp finely grated mozzarella cheese

For the cannoli filling:

- ½ cup ricotta cheese
- 2 tbsp swerve confectioner's sugar
- 1 tsp vanilla extract
- 2 tbsp unsweetened chocolate chips for garnishing

Directions:

1. Preheat the waffle iron.
2. Meanwhile, in a medium bowl, mix all the ingredients for the chaffles.
3. Open the iron, pour in a quarter of the mixture, cover, and cook until crispy, 7 minutes.
4. Remove the chaffle onto a plate and make 3 more with the remaining batter.
5. Meanwhile, for the cannoli filling:

6. Beat the ricotta cheese and swerve confectioner's sugar until smooth. Mix in the vanilla.
7. On each chaffle, spread some of the filling and wrap over.
8. Garnish the creamy ends with some chocolate chips.
9. Serve immediately.

Nutrition:

Calories 308

Fats 25.05g

Carbs 5.17g

Net Carbs 5.17g

Protein 15.18g

Nutter Butter Chaffles

Preparation Time: 15 minutes

Cooking Time: 14 minutes

Servings: 2

Ingredients:

For the chaffles:

- 2 tbsp sugar-free peanut butter powder
- 2 tbsp maple (sugar-free) syrup
- 1 egg, beaten
- ¼ cup finely grated mozzarella cheese
- ¼ tsp baking powder
- ¼ tsp almond butter
- ¼ tsp peanut butter extract
- 1 tbsp softened cream cheese

For the frosting:

- ½ cup almond flour
- 1 cup peanut butter
- 3 tbsp almond milk
- ½ tsp vanilla extract
- ½ cup maple (sugar-free) syrup

Directions:

1. Preheat the waffle iron.
2. Meanwhile, in a medium bowl, mix all the ingredients until smooth.
3. Open the iron and pour in half of the mixture.
4. Close the iron and cook until crispy, 6 to 7 minutes.

5. Remove the chaffle onto a plate and set aside.
6. Make a second chaffle with the remaining batter.
7. While the chaffles cool, make the frosting.
8. Pour the almond flour in a medium saucepan and stir-fry over medium heat until golden.
9. Transfer the almond flour to a blender and top with the remaining frosting ingredients. Process until smooth.
10. Spread the frosting on the chaffles and serve afterward.

Nutrition:

Calories 239

Fats 15.48g

Carbs 17.42g

Net Carbs 15.92g

Protein 7.52g

Chaffled Brownie Sundae

Preparation Time: 12 minutes

Cooking Time: 30 minutes

Servings: 4

Ingredients:

For the chaffles:

- 2 eggs, beaten
- 1 tbsp unsweetened cocoa powder
- 1 tbsp erythritol
- 1 cup finely grated mozzarella cheese

For the topping:

- 3 tbsp unsweetened chocolate, chopped
- 3 tbsp unsalted butter
- ½ cup swerve sugar
- Low-carb ice cream for topping
- 1 cup whipped cream for topping
- 3 tbsp sugar-free caramel sauce

Directions:

For the chaffles:

1. Preheat the waffle iron.
2. Meanwhile, in a medium bowl, mix all the ingredients for the chaffles.
3. Open the iron, pour in a quarter of the mixture, cover, and cook until crispy, 7 minutes.
4. Remove the chaffle onto a plate and make 3 more with the remaining batter.

5. Plate and set aside.

For the topping:

1. Meanwhile, melt the chocolate and butter in a medium saucepan with occasional stirring, 2 minutes.

To Servings:

1. Divide the chaffles into wedges and top with the ice cream, whipped cream, and swirl the chocolate sauce and caramel sauce on top.
2. Serve immediately.

<u>Nutrition:</u>

Calories 165

Fats 11.39g

Carbs 3.81g

Net Carbs 2.91g

Protein 12.79g

Brie and Blackberry Chaffles

Preparation Time: 15 minutes

Cooking Time: 36 minutes

Servings: 4

Ingredients:

For the chaffles:

- 2 eggs, beaten
- 1 cup finely grated mozzarella cheese
- For the topping:
- 1 ½ cups blackberries
- 1 lemon, 1 tsp zest and 2 tbsp juice
- 1 tbsp erythritol
- 4 slices Brie cheese

Directions:

For the chaffles:

1. Preheat the waffle iron.
2. Meanwhile, in a medium bowl, mix the eggs and mozzarella cheese.
3. Open the iron, pour in a quarter of the mixture, cover, and cook until crispy, 7 minutes.
4. Remove the chaffle onto a plate and make 3 more with the remaining batter.
5. Plate and set aside.

For the topping:

1. In a medium pot, add the blackberries, lemon zest, lemon juice, and erythritol. Cook until the blackberries break and the sauce thickens, 5 minutes. Turn the heat off.
2. Arrange the chaffles on the baking sheet and place two Brie cheese slices on each. Top with blackberry mixture and transfer the baking sheet to the oven.
3. Bake until the cheese melts, 2 to 3 minutes.
4. Remove from the oven, allow cooling and serve afterward.

Nutrition:

Calories 576

Fats 42.22g

Carbs 7.07g

Net Carbs 3.67g

Protein 42.35g

Cereal Chaffle Cake

Preparation Time: 5 minutes

Cooking Time: 8 minutes

Servings: 2

Ingredients:

- 1 egg
- 2 tablespoons almond flour
- ½ teaspoon coconut flour
- 1 tablespoon melted butter
- 1 tablespoon cream cheese
- 1 tablespoon plain cereal, crushed
- ¼ teaspoon vanilla extract
- ¼ teaspoon baking powder
- 1 tablespoon sweetener
- 1/8 teaspoon xanthan gum

Directions:

1. Plug in your waffle maker to preheat.
2. Add all the ingredients in a large bowl.
3. Mix until well blended.
4. Let the batter rest for 2 minutes before cooking.
5. Pour half of the mixture into the waffle maker.
6. Seal and cook for 4 minutes.
7. Make the next chaffle using the same steps.

Nutrition:

Calories154

Total Fat 21.2g

Saturated Fat 10 g

Cholesterol 113.3mg

Sodium 96.9mg

Potassium 453 mg

Total Carbohydrate 5.9g

Dietary Fiber 1.7g

Protein 4.6g

Total Sugars 2.7g

Ham, Cheese & Tomato Chaffle Sandwich

Preparation Time: 5 minutes

Cooking Time: 10 minutes

Servings: 2

Ingredients:

- 1 teaspoon olive oil
- 2 slices ham
- 4 basic chaffles
- 1 tablespoon mayonnaise
- 2 slices Provolone cheese
- 1 tomato, sliced

Directions:

1. Add the olive oil to a pan over medium heat.
2. Cook the ham for 1 minute per side.
3. Spread the chaffles with mayonnaise.
4. Top with the ham, cheese and tomatoes.
5. Top with another chaffle to make a sandwich.

Nutrition:

Calories 198

Total Fat 14.7g

Saturated Fat 6.3g

Cholesterol 37mg

Sodium 664mg

Total Carbohydrate 4.6g

Dietary Fiber 0.7g

Total Sugars 1.5g

Protein 12.2g

Potassium 193mg

Broccoli & Cheese Chaffle

Preparation Time: 5 minutes

Cooking Time: 8 minutes

Servings: 2

Ingredients:

- ¼ cup broccoli florets
- 1 egg, beaten
- 1 tablespoon almond flour
- ¼ teaspoon garlic powder
- ½ cup cheddar cheese

Directions:

1. Preheat your waffle maker.
2. Add the broccoli to the food processor.
3. Pulse until chopped.
4. Add to a bowl.
5. Stir in the egg and the rest of the ingredients.
6. Mix well.
7. Pour half of the batter to the waffle maker.
8. Cover and cook for 4 minutes.
9. Repeat procedure to make the next chaffle.

Nutrition:

Calories 170

Total Fat 13 g

Saturated Fat 7 g

Cholesterol 112 mg

Sodium 211 mg

Potassium 94 mg

Total Carbohydrate 2 g

Dietary Fiber 1 g

Protein 11 g

Total Sugars 1 g

Carrot Chaffle Cake

Preparation Time: 15 minutes

Cooking Time: 24 minutes

Servings: 6

Ingredients:

- 1 egg, beaten
- 2 tablespoons melted butter
- ½ cup carrot, shredded
- ¾ cup almond flour
- 1 teaspoon baking powder
- 2 tablespoons heavy whipping cream
- 2 tablespoons sweetener
- 1 tablespoon walnuts, chopped
- 1 teaspoon pumpkin spice
- 2 teaspoons cinnamon

Directions:

1. Preheat your waffle maker.
2. In a large bowl, combine all the ingredients.
3. Pour some of the mixture into the waffle maker.
4. Close and cook for 4 minutes.
5. Repeat steps until all the remaining batter has been used.

Nutrition:

Calories 294

Total Fat 26.7g

Saturated Fat 12g

Cholesterol 133mg

Sodium 144mg

Potassium 421mg

Total Carbohydrate 11.6g

Dietary Fiber 4.5g

Protein 6.8g

Total Sugars 1.7g

Chaffle with Sausage Gravy

Preparation Time: 5 minutes

Cooking Time: 15 minutes

Servings: 2

Ingredients:

- ¼ cup sausage, cooked
- 3 tablespoons chicken broth
- 2 teaspoons cream cheese
- 2 tablespoons heavy whipping cream
- ¼ teaspoon garlic powder
- Pepper to taste
- 2 basic chaffles

Directions:

1. Add the sausage, broth, cream cheese, cream, garlic powder and pepper to a pan over medium heat.
2. Bring to a boil and then reduce heat.
3. Simmer for 10 minutes or until the sauce has thickened.
4. Pour the gravy on top of the basic chaffles
5. Serve.

Nutrition:

Calories 212

Total Fat 17 g

Saturated Fat 10 g

Cholesterol 134 mg

Sodium 350 mg

Potassium 133 mg

Total Carbohydrate 3 g

Dietary Fiber 1 g

Protein 11 g

Total Sugars 1 g

Barbecue Chaffle

Preparation Time: 5 minutes

Cooking Time: 8 minutes

Servings: 2

Ingredients:

- 1 egg, beaten
- ½ cup cheddar cheese, shredded
- ½ teaspoon barbecue sauce
- ¼ teaspoon baking powder

Directions:

1. Plug in your waffle maker to preheat.
2. Mix all the ingredients in a bowl.
3. Pour half of the mixture to your waffle maker.
4. Cover and cook for 4 minutes.
5. Repeat the same steps for the next barbecue chaffle.

Nutrition:

Calories 295

Total Fat 23 g

Saturated Fat 13 g

Cholesterol 223 mg

Sodium 414 mg

Potassium 179 mg

Total Carbohydrate 2 g

Dietary Fiber 1 g

Protein 20 g

Total Sugars 1 g

Pumpkin & Pecan Chaffle

Preparation Time: 5 minutes

Cooking Time: 10 minutes

Servings: 2

Ingredients:

- 1 egg, beaten
- ½ cup mozzarella cheese, grated
- ½ teaspoon pumpkin spice
- 1 tablespoon pureed pumpkin
- 2 tablespoons almond flour
- 1 teaspoon sweetener
- 2 tablespoons pecans, chopped

Directions:

1. Turn on the waffle maker.
2. Beat the egg in a bowl.
3. Stir in the rest of the ingredients.
4. Pour half of the mixture into the device.
5. Seal the lid.
6. Cook for 5 minutes.
7. Remove the chaffle carefully.
8. Repeat the steps to make the second chaffle.

Nutrition:

Calories 210

Total Fat 17 g

Saturated Fat 10 g

Cholesterol 110 mg

Sodium 250 mg

Potassium 570 mg

Total Carbohydrate 4.6 g

Dietary Fiber 1.7 g

Protein 11 g

Total Sugars 2 g

Double Choco Chaffle

Preparation Time: 5 minutes

Cooking Time: 10 minutes

Servings: 2

Ingredients:

- 1 egg
- 2 teaspoons coconut flour
- 2 tablespoons sweetener
- 1 tablespoon cocoa powder
- ¼ teaspoon baking powder
- 1 oz. cream cheese
- ½ teaspoon vanilla
- 1 tablespoon sugar-free chocolate chips

Directions:

1. Put all the ingredients in a large bowl.
2. Mix well.
3. Pour half of the mixture into the waffle maker.
4. Seal the device.
5. Cook for 4 minutes.
6. Uncover and transfer to a plate to cool.
7. Repeat the procedure to make the second chaffle.

Nutrition:

Calories 171

Total Fat 10.7g

Saturated Fat 5.3g

Cholesterol 97mg

Sodium 106mg

Potassium 179mg

Total Carbohydrate 3g

Dietary Fiber 4.8g

Protein 5.8g

Total Sugars 0.4g

Cream Cheese Chaffle

Preparation Time: 5 minutes

Cooking Time: 8 minutes

Servings: 2

Ingredients:

- 1 egg, beaten
- 1 oz. cream cheese
- ½ teaspoon vanilla
- 4 teaspoons sweetener
- ¼ teaspoon baking powder
- Cream cheese

Directions:

1. Preheat your waffle maker.
2. Add all the ingredients in a bowl.
3. Mix well.
4. Pour half of the batter into the waffle maker.
5. Seal the device.
6. Cook for 4 minutes.
7. Remove the chaffle from the waffle maker.
8. Make the second one using the same steps.
9. Spread remaining cream cheese on top before serving.

Nutrition:

Calories 169

Total Fat 14.3g

Saturated Fat 7.6g

Cholesterol 195mg

Sodium 147mg

Potassium 222mg

Total Carbohydrate 4g

Dietary Fiber 4g

Protein 7.7g

Total Sugars 0.7g

Bacon & Chicken Ranch Chaffle

Preparation Time: 5 minutes

Cooking Time: 8 minutes

Servings: 2

Ingredients:

- 1 egg
- ¼ cup chicken cubes, cooked
- 1 slice bacon, cooked and chopped
- ¼ cup cheddar cheese, shredded
- 1 teaspoon ranch dressing powder

Directions:

1. Preheat your waffle maker.
2. In a bowl, mix all the ingredients.
3. Add half of the mixture to your waffle maker.
4. Cover and cook for 4 minutes.
5. Make the second chaffle using the same steps.

Nutrition:

Calories 200

Total Fat 14 g

Saturated Fat 6 g

Cholesterol 129 mg

Sodium 463 mg

Potassium 130 mg

Total Carbohydrate 2 g

Dietary Fiber 1 g

Protein 16 g

Total Sugars 1 g

Cheeseburger Chaffle

Preparation Time: 15 minutes

Cooking Time: 15 minutes

Servings: 2

Ingredients:

- 1 lb. ground beef
- 1 onion, minced
- 1 tsp. parsley, chopped
- 1 egg, beaten
- Salt and pepper to taste
- 1 tablespoon olive oil
- 4 basic chaffles
- 2 lettuce leaves
- 2 cheese slices
- 1 tablespoon dill pickles
- Ketchup
- Mayonnaise

Directions:

1. In a large bowl, combine the ground beef, onion, parsley, egg, salt and pepper.
2. Mix well.
3. Form 2 thick patties.
4. Add olive oil to the pan.
5. Place the pan over medium heat.
6. Cook the patty for 3 to 5 minutes per side or until fully cooked.
7. Place the patty on top of each chaffle.

8. Top with lettuce, cheese and pickles.
9. Squirt ketchup and mayo over the patty and veggies.
10. Top with another chaffle.

Nutrition:

Calories 325

Total Fat 16.3g

Saturated Fat 6.5g

Cholesterol 157mg

Sodium 208mg

Total Carbohydrate 3g

Dietary Fiber 0.7g

Total Sugars 1.4g

Protein 39.6g

Potassium 532mg

Intermediate

Chaffle Fruit Snacks

Preparation Time: 10 minutes

Cooking Time: 14 minutes

Servings: 2

Ingredients:

- 1 egg, beaten
- ½ cup finely grated cheddar cheese
- ½ cup Greek yogurt for topping
- 8 raspberries and blackberries for topping

Directions:

1. Preheat the waffle iron.
2. Mix the egg and cheddar cheese in a medium bowl.
3. Open the iron and add half of the mixture. Close and cook until crispy, 7 minutes.
4. Remove the chaffle onto a plate and make another with the remaining mixture.
5. Cut each chaffle into wedges and arrange on a plate.
6. Top each waffle with a tablespoon of yogurt and then two berries.
7. Serve afterward.

Nutrition:

Calories 207

Fats 15.29g

Carbs 4.36g

Net Carbs 3.86g

Protein 12.91g

Keto Belgian Sugar Chaffles

Preparation Time: 10 minutes

Cooking Time: 24 minutes

Servings: 4

Ingredients:

- 1 egg, beaten
- 2 tbsp swerve brown sugar
- ½ tbsp butter, melted
- 1 tsp vanilla extract
- 1 cup finely grated Parmesan cheese

Directions:

1. Preheat the waffle iron.
2. Mix all the ingredients in a medium bowl.
3. Open the iron and pour in a quarter of the mixture. Close and cook until crispy, 6 minutes.
4. Remove the chaffle onto a plate and make 3 more with the remaining ingredients.
5. Cut each chaffle into wedges, plate, allow cooling and serve.

Nutrition:

Calories 136

Net Carbs 3.69g

Fats 9.45g

Protein 8.5g

Carbs 3.69g

Lemon and Paprika Chaffles

Preparation Time: 10 minutes

Cooking Time: 28 minutes

Servings: 4

Ingredients:

- 1 egg, beaten
- 1 oz cream cheese, softened
- 1/3 cup finely grated mozzarella cheese
- 1 tbsp almond flour
- 1 tsp butter, melted
- 1 tsp maple (sugar-free) syrup
- ½ tsp sweet paprika
- ½ tsp lemon extract

Directions:

1. Preheat the waffle iron.
2. Mix all the ingredients in a medium bowl
3. Open the iron and pour in a quarter of the mixture. Close and cook until crispy, 7 minutes.
4. Remove the chaffle onto a plate and make 3 more with the remaining mixture.
5. Cut each chaffle into wedges, plate, allow cooling and serve.

Nutrition:

Calories 48

Fats 4.22g

Carbs 0.6g

Net Carbs 0.5g

Protein 2g

Pumpkin Spice Chaffles

Preparation Time: 10 minutes

Cooking Time: 14 minutes

Servings: 2

Ingredients:

- 1 egg, beaten
- ½ tsp pumpkin pie spice
- ½ cup finely grated mozzarella cheese
- 1 tbsp sugar-free pumpkin puree

Directions:

1. Preheat the waffle iron.
2. In a medium bowl, mix all the ingredients.
3. Open the iron, pour in half of the batter, close, and cook until crispy, 6 to 7 minutes.
4. Remove the chaffle onto a plate and set aside.
5. Make another chaffle with the remaining batter.
6. Allow cooling and serve afterward.

Nutrition:

Calories 90

Fats 6.46g

Carbs 1.98g

Net Carbs 1.58g

Protein 5.94g

Breakfast Spinach Ricotta Chaffles

Preparation Time: 10 minutes

Cooking Time: 28 minutes

Servings: 4

Ingredients:

- 4 oz frozen spinach, thawed, squeezed dry
- 1 cup ricotta cheese
- 2 eggs, beaten
- ½ tsp garlic powder
- ¼ cup finely grated Pecorino Romano cheese
- ½ cup finely grated mozzarella cheese
- Salt and freshly ground black pepper to taste

Directions:

1. Preheat the waffle iron.
2. In a medium bowl, mix all the ingredients.
3. Open the iron, lightly grease with cooking spray and spoon in a quarter of the mixture.
4. Close the iron and cook until brown and crispy, 7 minutes.
5. Remove the chaffle onto a plate and set aside.
6. Make three more chaffles with the remaining mixture.
7. Allow cooling and serve afterward.

Nutrition:

Calories 188

Fats 13.15g

Carbs 5.06g

Net Carbs 4.06g

Protein 12.79g

Scrambled Egg Stuffed Chaffles

Preparation Time: 15 minutes

Cooking Time: 28 minutes

Servings: 4

Ingredients:

For the chaffles:

- 1 cup finely grated cheddar cheese
- 2 eggs, beaten
- For the egg stuffing:
- 1 tbsp olive oil
- 1 small red bell pepper
- 4 large eggs
- 1 small green bell pepper
- Salt and freshly ground black pepper to taste
- 2 tbsp grated Parmesan cheese

Directions:

For the chaffles:

1. Preheat the waffle iron.
2. In a medium bowl, mix the cheddar cheese and egg.
3. Open the iron, pour in a quarter of the mixture, close, and cook until crispy, 6 to 7 minutes.
4. Plate and make three more chaffles using the remaining mixture.

For the egg stuffing:

1. Meanwhile, heat the olive oil in a medium skillet over medium heat on a stovetop.

2. In a medium bowl, beat the eggs with the bell peppers, salt, black pepper, and Parmesan cheese.
3. Pour the mixture into the skillet and scramble until set to your likeness, 2 minutes.
4. Between two chaffles, spoon half of the scrambled eggs and repeat with the second set of chaffles.
5. Serve afterward.

Nutrition Facts per Serving:

Calories 387

Fats 22.52g

Carbs 18.12g

Net Carbs 17.52g

Protein 27.76g

Herby Chaffle Snacks

Preparation Time: 10 minutes

Cooking Time: 28 minutes

Servings: 4

Ingredients:

- 1 egg, beaten
- ½ cup finely grated Monterey Jack cheese
- ¼ cup finely grated Parmesan cheese
- ½ tsp dried mixed herbs

Directions:

1. Preheat the waffle iron.
2. Mix all the ingredients in a medium bowl
3. Open the iron and pour in a quarter of the mixture. Close and cook until crispy, 7 minutes.
4. Remove the chaffle onto a plate and make 3 more with the rest of the ingredients.
5. Cut each chaffle into wedges and plate.
6. Allow cooling and serve.

Nutrition:

Calories 96

Fats 6.29g

Carbs 2.19g

Net Carbs 2.19g

Protein 7.42g

Ham and Cheddar Chaffles

Preparation Time: 15 minutes

Cooking Time: 28 minutes

Servings: 4

Ingredients:

- 1 cup finely shredded parsnips, steamed
- 8 oz ham, diced
- 2 eggs, beaten
- 1 ½ cups finely grated cheddar cheese
- ½ tsp garlic powder
- 2 tbsp chopped fresh parsley leaves
- ¼ tsp smoked paprika
- ½ tsp dried thyme
- Salt and freshly ground black pepper to taste

Directions:

1. Preheat the waffle iron.
2. In a medium bowl, mix all the ingredients.
3. Open the iron, lightly grease with cooking spray and pour in a quarter of the mixture.
4. Close the iron and cook until crispy, 7 minutes.
5. Remove the chaffle onto a plate and set aside.
6. Make three more chaffles using the remaining mixture.
7. Serve afterward.

Nutrition Facts per Serving:

Calories 506

Fats 24.05g

Carbs 30.02g

Net Carbs 28.22g

Protein 42.74g

Savory Gruyere and Chives Chaffles

Preparation Time: 15 minutes

Cooking Time: 14 minutes

Servings: 2

Ingredients:

- 2 eggs, beaten
- 1 cup finely grated Gruyere cheese
- 2 tbsp finely grated cheddar cheese
- 1/8 tsp freshly ground black pepper
- 3 tbsp minced fresh chives + more for garnishing
- 2 sunshine fried eggs for topping

Directions:

1. Preheat the waffle iron.
2. In a medium bowl, mix the eggs, cheeses, black pepper, and chives.
3. Open the iron and pour in half of the mixture.
4. Close the iron and cook until brown and crispy, 7 minutes.
5. Remove the chaffle onto a plate and set aside.
6. Make another chaffle using the remaining mixture.
7. Top each chaffle with one fried egg each, garnish with the chives and serve.

Nutrition Facts per Serving:

Calories 712

Net Carbs 3.78g

Fats 41.32g

Protein 23.75g

Carbs 3.88g

Chicken Quesadilla Chaffle

Preparation Time: 10 minutes

Cooking Time: 14 minutes

Servings: 2

Ingredients:

- 1 egg, beaten
- ¼ tsp taco seasoning
- 1/3 cup finely grated cheddar cheese
- 1/3 cup cooked chopped chicken

Directions:

1. Preheat the waffle iron.
2. In a medium bowl, mix the eggs, taco seasoning, and cheddar cheese. Add the chicken and combine well.
3. Open the iron, lightly grease with cooking spray and pour in half of the mixture.
4. Close the iron and cook until brown and crispy, 7 minutes.
5. Remove the chaffle onto a plate and set aside.
6. Make another chaffle using the remaining mixture.
7. Serve afterward.

Nutrition Facts per Serving:

Calories 314

Fats 20.64g

Carbs 5.71g

Net Carbs 5.71g

Protein 16.74g

Mixed Berry-Vanilla Chaffles

Preparation Time: 10 minutes

Cooking Time: 28 minutes

Servings: 4

Ingredients:

- 1 egg, beaten
- ½ cup finely grated mozzarella cheese
- 1 tbsp cream cheese, softened
- 1 tbsp sugar-free maple syrup
- 2 strawberries, sliced
- 2 raspberries, slices
- ¼ tsp blackberry extract
- ¼ tsp vanilla extract
- ½ cup plain yogurt for serving

Directions:

1. Preheat the waffle iron.
2. In a medium bowl, mix all the ingredients except the yogurt.
3. Open the iron, lightly grease with cooking spray and pour in a quarter of the mixture.
4. Close the iron and cook until golden brown and crispy, 7 minutes.
5. Remove the chaffle onto a plate and set aside.
6. Make three more chaffles with the remaining mixture.
7. To Servings: top with the yogurt and enjoy.

Nutrition Facts per Serving:

Calories 78

Fats 5.29g

Carbs 3.02g

Net Carbs 2.72g

Protein 4.32g

Hot Chocolate Breakfast Chaffle

Preparation Time: 10 minutes

Cooking Time: 14 minutes

Servings: 2

Ingredients:

- 1 egg, beaten
- 2 tbsp almond flour
- 1 tbsp unsweetened cocoa powder
- 2 tbsp cream cheese, softened
- ¼ cup finely grated Monterey Jack cheese
- 2 tbsp sugar-free maple syrup
- 1 tsp vanilla extract

Directions:

1. Preheat the waffle iron.
2. In a medium bowl, mix all the ingredients.
3. Open the iron, lightly grease with cooking spray and pour in half of the mixture.
4. Close the iron and cook until crispy, 7 minutes.
5. Remove the chaffle onto a plate and set aside.
6. Pour the remaining batter in the iron and make the second chaffle.
7. Allow cooling and serve afterward.

Nutrition Facts per Serving:

Calories 47

Net Carbs 0.89g

Fats 3.67g

Protein 2.29g

Carbs 1.39g

Blueberry Chaffles

Preparation Time: 15 minutes

Servings: 4

Ingredients:

- 2 eggs
- 1/2 cup blueberries
- 1/2 tsp baking powder
- 1/2 tsp vanilla
- 2 tsp Swerve
- 3 tbsp almond flour
- 1 cup mozzarella cheese, shredded

Directions:

1. Preheat your waffle maker.
2. In a medium bowl, mix eggs, vanilla, Swerve, almond flour, and cheese.
3. Add blueberries and stir well.
4. Spray waffle maker with cooking spray.
5. Pour 1/4 batter in the hot waffle maker and cook for 5-8 minutes or until golden brown. Repeat with the remaining batter.
6. Serve and enjoy.

Nutrition:

Calories 96

Fat 6.1 g

Carbohydrates 5.7 g

Sugar 2.2 g

Protein 6.1 g

Cholesterol 86 mg

Pumpkin Cheesecake Chaffle

Preparation Time: 15 minutes

Servings: 2

Ingredients:

For chaffle:

- 1 egg
- 1/2 tsp vanilla
- 1/2 tsp baking powder, gluten-free
- 1/4 tsp pumpkin spice
- 1 tsp cream cheese, softened
- 2 tsp heavy cream
- 1 tbsp Swerve
- 1 tbsp almond flour
- 2 tsp pumpkin puree
- 1/2 cup mozzarella cheese, shredded

For filling:

- 1/4 tsp vanilla
- 1 tbsp Swerve
- 2 tbsp cream cheese

Directions:

1. Preheat your mini waffle maker.
2. In a small bowl, mix all chaffle ingredients.
3. Spray waffle maker with cooking spray.
4. Pour half batter in the hot waffle maker and cook for 3-5 minutes. Repeat with the remaining batter.
5. In a small bowl, combine all filling ingredients.

6. Spread filling mixture between two chaffles and place in the fridge for 10 minutes.
7. Serve and enjoy.

<u>Nutrition:</u>

Calories 107

Fat 7.2 g

Carbohydrates 5 g

Sugar 0.7 g

Protein 6.7 g

Cholesterol 93 mg

Quick & Easy Blueberry Chaffle

Preparation Time: 15 minutes

Servings: 2

Ingredients:

- 1 egg, lightly beaten
- 1/4 cup blueberries
- 1/2 tsp vanilla
- 1 oz cream cheese
- 1/4 tsp baking powder, gluten-free
- 4 tsp Swerve
- 1 tbsp coconut flour

Directions:

1. Preheat your waffle maker.
2. In a small bowl, mix coconut flour, baking powder, and Swerve until well combined.
3. Add vanilla, cream cheese, egg, and vanilla and whisk until combined.
4. Spray waffle maker with cooking spray.
5. Pour half batter in the hot waffle maker and top with 4-5 blueberries and cook for 4-5 minutes until golden brown. Repeat with the remaining batter.
6. Serve and enjoy.

Nutrition:

Calories 135

Fat 8.2 g

Carbohydrates 11 g

Sugar 2.6 g

Protein 5 g

Cholesterol 97 mg

Pecan Pumpkin Chaffle

Preparation Time: 15 minutes

Servings: 2

Ingredients:

- 1 egg
- 2 tbsp pecans, toasted and chopped
- 2 tbsp almond flour
- 1 tsp erythritol
- 1/4 tsp pumpkin pie spice
- 1 tbsp pumpkin puree
- 1/2 cup mozzarella cheese, grated

Directions:

1. Preheat your waffle maker.
2. Beat egg in a small bowl.
3. Add remaining ingredients and mix well.
4. Spray waffle maker with cooking spray.
5. Pour half batter in the hot waffle maker and cook for 5 minutes or until golden brown. Repeat with the remaining batter.
6. Serve and enjoy.

<u>Nutrition:</u>

Calories 121

Fat 9.7 g

Carbohydrates 5.7 g

Sugar 3.3 g

Protein 6.7 g

Cholesterol 86 mg

Cinnamon Cream Cheese Chaffle

Preparation Time: 15 minutes

Servings: 2

Ingredients:

- 2 eggs, lightly beaten
- 1 tsp collagen
- ¼ tsp baking powder, gluten-free
- 1 tsp monk fruit sweetener
- ½ tsp cinnamon
- ¼ cup cream cheese, softened
- Pinch of salt

Directions:

1. Preheat your waffle maker.
2. Add all ingredients into the bowl and beat using hand mixer until well combined.
3. Spray waffle maker with cooking spray.
4. Pour 1/2 batter in the hot waffle maker and cook for 3-4 minutes or until golden brown. Repeat with the remaining batter.
5. Serve and enjoy.

Nutrition:

Calories 179

Sugar 0.4 g

Fat 14.5 g

Protein 10.8 g

Carbohydrates 1.9 g

Cholesterol 196 mg

Mozzarella Peanut Butter Chaffle

Preparation Time: 15 minutes

Servings: 2

Ingredients:

- 1 egg, lightly beaten
- 2 tbsp peanut butter
- 2 tbsp Swerve
- 1/2 cup mozzarella cheese, shredded

Directions:

1. Preheat your waffle maker.
2. In a bowl, mix egg, cheese, Swerve, and peanut butter until well combined.
3. Spray waffle maker with cooking spray.
4. Pour half batter in the hot waffle maker and cook for 4 minutes or until golden brown. Repeat with the remaining batter.
5. Serve and enjoy.

Nutrition:

Calories 150

Fat 11.5 g

Carbohydrates 5.6 g

Sugar 1.7 g

Protein 8.8 g

Cholesterol 86 mg

Apple Cinnamon Chaffles

Preparation Time: 20 minutes

Servings: 3

Ingredients:

- 3 eggs, lightly beaten
- 1 cup mozzarella cheese, shredded
- ¼ cup apple, chopped
- ½ tsp monk fruit sweetener
- 1 ½ tsp cinnamon
- ¼ tsp baking powder, gluten-free
- 2 tbsp coconut flour

Directions:

1. Preheat your waffle maker.
2. Add remaining ingredients and stir until well combined.
3. Spray waffle maker with cooking spray.
4. Pour 1/3 of batter in the hot waffle maker and cook for 4 minutes or until golden brown. Repeat with the remaining batter.
5. Serve and enjoy.

<u>Nutrition:</u>

Calories 142

Fat 7.4 g

Carbohydrates 9.7 g

Sugar 3 g

Protein 9.6 g

Cholesterol 169 mg

Choco Chip Pumpkin Chaffle

Preparation Time: 15 minutes

Servings: 2

Ingredients:

- 1 egg, lightly beaten
- 1 tbsp almond flour
- 1 tbsp unsweetened chocolate chips
- 1/4 tsp pumpkin pie spice
- 2 tbsp Swerve
- 1 tbsp pumpkin puree
- 1/2 cup mozzarella cheese, shredded

Directions:

1. Preheat your waffle maker.
2. In a small bowl, mix egg and pumpkin puree.
3. Add pumpkin pie spice, Swerve, almond flour, and cheese and mix well.
4. Stir in chocolate chips.
5. Spray waffle maker with cooking spray.
6. Pour half batter in the hot waffle maker and cook for 4 minutes. Repeat with the remaining batter.
7. Serve and enjoy.

Nutrition:

Calories 130

Fat 9.2 g

Carbohydrates 5.9 g

Sugar 0.6 g

Protein 6.6 g

Cholesterol 86 mg

Maple Chaffle

Preparation Time: 15 minutes

Servings: 2

<u>Ingredients:</u>

- 1 egg, lightly beaten
- 2 egg whites
- 1/2 tsp maple extract
- 2 tsp Swerve
- 1/2 tsp baking powder, gluten-free
- 2 tbsp almond milk
- 2 tbsp coconut flour

<u>Directions:</u>

1. Preheat your waffle maker.
2. In a bowl, whip egg whites until stiff peaks form.
3. Stir in maple extract, Swerve, baking powder, almond milk, coconut flour, and egg.
4. Spray waffle maker with cooking spray.
5. Pour half batter in the hot waffle maker and cook for 3-5 minutes or until golden brown. Repeat with the remaining batter.
6. Serve and enjoy.

Nutrition:

Calories 122

Fat 6.6 g

Carbohydrates 9 g

Sugar 1 g

Protein 7.7 g

Cholesterol 82 mg

Peanut Butter Sandwich Chaffle

Preparation Time: 15 minutes

Servings: 1

Ingredients:

For chaffle:

- 1 egg, lightly beaten
- 1/2 cup mozzarella cheese, shredded
- 1/4 tsp espresso powder
- 1 tbsp unsweetened chocolate chips
- 1 tbsp Swerve
- 2 tbsp unsweetened cocoa powder

For filling:

- 1 tbsp butter, softened
- 2 tbsp Swerve
- 3 tbsp creamy peanut butter

Directions:

1. Preheat your waffle maker.
2. In a bowl, whisk together egg, espresso powder, chocolate chips, Swerve, and cocoa powder.
3. Add mozzarella cheese and stir well.
4. Spray waffle maker with cooking spray.
5. Pour 1/2 of the batter in the hot waffle maker and cook for 3-4 minutes or until golden brown. Repeat with the remaining batter.
6. For filling: In a small bowl, stir together butter, Swerve, and peanut butter until smooth.

7. Once chaffles is cool, then spread filling mixture between two chaffle and place in the fridge for 10 minutes.
8. Cut chaffle sandwich in half and serve.

Nutrition:

Calories 190

Fat 16.1 g

Carbohydrates 9.6 g

Sugar 1.1 g

Protein 8.2 g

Cholesterol 101 mg

Cherry Chocolate Chaffle

Preparation Time: 10 minutes

Servings: 1

Ingredients:

- 1 egg, lightly beaten
- 1 tbsp unsweetened chocolate chips
- 2 tbsp sugar-free cherry pie filling
- 2 tbsp heavy whipping cream
- 1/2 cup mozzarella cheese, shredded
- 1/2 tsp baking powder, gluten-free
- 1 tbsp Swerve
- 1 tbsp unsweetened cocoa powder
- 1 tbsp almond flour

Directions:

1. Preheat the waffle maker.
2. In a bowl, whisk together egg, cheese, baking powder, Swerve, cocoa powder, and almond flour.
3. Spray waffle maker with cooking spray.
4. Pour batter in the hot waffle maker and cook until golden brown.
5. Top with cherry pie filling, heavy whipping cream, and chocolate chips and serve.

Nutrition:

Calories 264

Fat 22 g

Carbohydrates 8.5 g

Sugar 0.5 g

Protein 12.7 g

Cholesterol 212 mg

Choco Chip Lemon Chaffle

Preparation Time: 15 minutes

Servings: 2

Ingredients:

- 2 eggs, lightly beaten
- 1 tbsp unsweetened chocolate chips
- 2 tsp Swerve
- 1/2 tsp vanilla
- 1/2 tsp lemon extract
- 1/2 cup mozzarella cheese, shredded
- 2 tsp almond flour

Directions:

1. Preheat your waffle maker.
2. In a bowl, whisk eggs, Swerve, vanilla, lemon extract, cheese, and almond flour.
3. Add chocolate chips and stir well.
4. Spray waffle maker with cooking spray.
5. Pour 1/2 of the batter in the hot waffle maker and cook for 4-5 minutes or until golden brown. Repeat with the remaining batter.
6. Serve and enjoy.

Nutrition:

Calories 157

Fat 10.8 g

Carbohydrates 5.4 g

Sugar 0.7 g

Protein 9 g

Cholesterol 167 mg

Sweet Vanilla Chocolate Chaffle

Preparation Time: 10 minutes

Servings: 1

Ingredients:

- 1 egg, lightly beaten
- 1/4 tsp cinnamon
- 1/2 tsp vanilla
- 1 tbsp Swerve
- 2 tsp unsweetened cocoa powder
- 1 tbsp coconut flour
- 2 oz cream cheese, softened

Directions:

1. Add all ingredients into the small bowl and mix until well combined.
2. Spray waffle maker with cooking spray.
3. Pour batter in the hot waffle maker and cook until golden brown.
4. Serve and enjoy.

Nutrition:

Calories 312

Fat 25.4 g

Carbohydrates 11.5 g

Sugar 0.8 g

Protein 11.6 g

Cholesterol 226 mg

Expert

Bacon, Egg & Avocado Chaffle Sandwich

Preparation Time: 5 minutes

Cooking Time: 10 minutes

Servings: 2

Ingredients:

- Cooking spray
- 4 slices bacon
- 2 eggs
- ½ avocado, mashed
- 4 basic chaffles
- 2 leaves lettuce

Method:

1. Coat your skillet with cooking spray.
2. Cook the bacon until golden and crisp.
3. Transfer into a paper towel lined plate.
4. Crack the eggs into the same pan and cook until firm.
5. Flip and cook until the yolk is set.
6. Spread the avocado on the chaffle.
7. Top with lettuce, egg and bacon.
8. Top with another chaffle.

Nutritional Value:

- Calories 372
- Total Fat 30.1g
- Saturated Fat 8.6g
- Cholesterol 205mg
- Sodium 943mg
- Total Carbohydrate 5.4g
- Dietary Fiber 3.4g
- Total Sugars 0.6g
- Protein 20.6g
- Potassium 524mg

Pumpkin Chaffles with Choco Chips

Preparation Time: 5 minutes

Cooking Time: 12 minutes

Servings: 3

Ingredients:

- 1 egg
- ½ cup shredded mozzarella cheese
- 4 teaspoons pureed pumpkin
- ¼ teaspoon pumpkin pie spice
- 2 tablespoons sweetener
- 1 tablespoon almond flour
- 4 teaspoons chocolate chips (sugar-free)

Method:

1. Turn your waffle maker on.
2. In a bowl, beat the egg and stir in the pureed pumpkin.
3. Mix well.
4. Add the rest of the ingredients one by one.
5. Pour 1/3 of the mixture to your waffle maker.
6. Cook for 4 minutes.
7. Repeat the same steps with the remaining mixture.

Nutritional Value:

- Calories 93
- Total Fat 7 g
- Saturated Fat 3 g
- Cholesterol 69 mg
- Sodium 138 mg
- Potassium 48 mg
- Total Carbohydrate 2 g
- Dietary Fiber 1 g
- Protein 7 g
- Total Sugars 1 g

Open-Faced Ham & Green Bell Pepper Chaffle Sandwich

Preparation Time: 10 minutes

Cooking Time: 10 minutes

Servings: 2

Ingredients:

- 2 slices ham
- Cooking spray
- 1 green bell pepper, sliced into strips
- 2 slices cheese
- 1 tablespoon black olives, pitted and sliced
- 2 basic chaffles

Method:

1. Cook the ham in a pan coated with oil over medium heat.
2. Next, cook the bell pepper.
3. Assemble the open-faced sandwich by topping each chaffle with ham and cheese, bell pepper and olives.
4. Toast in the oven until the cheese has melted a little.

Nutritional Value:

- Calories 365
- Total Fat 24.6g
- Saturated Fat 13.6g
- Cholesterol 91mg
- Sodium 1154mg
- Potassium 440mg
- Total Carbohydrate 8g
- Dietary Fiber 2.6g
- Protein 24.5g
- Total Sugars 6.3g

Mini Keto Pizza

Preparation Time: 10 minutes

Cooking Time: 15 minutes

Servings: 2

Ingredients:

- 1 egg
- ½ cup mozzarella cheese, shredded
- ¼ teaspoon basil
- ¼ teaspoon garlic powder
- 1 tablespoon almond flour
- ½ teaspoon baking powder
- 2 tablespoons reduced-carb pasta sauce
- 2 tablespoons mozzarella cheese

Method:

1. Preheat your waffle maker.
2. In a bowl, beat the egg.
3. Stir in the ½ cup mozzarella cheese, basil, garlic powder, almond flour and baking powder.
4. Add half of the mixture to your waffle maker.
5. Cook for 4 minutes.
6. Transfer to a baking sheet.
7. Cook the second mini pizza.
8. While both pizzas are on the baking sheet, spread the pasta sauce on top.
9. Sprinkle the cheese on top.
10. Bake in the oven until the cheese has melted.

Nutritional Value:

- Calories 195
- Total Fat 14 g
- Saturated Fat 6 g
- Cholesterol 116 mg
- Sodium 301 mg
- Potassium 178 mg
- Total Carbohydrate 4 g
- Dietary Fiber 1 g
- Protein 13 g
- Total Sugars 1 g

Pumkpin Chaffle with Maple Syrup

Preparation Time: 5 minutes

Cooking Time: 16 minutes

Servings: 2

Ingredients:

- 2 eggs, beaten
- ½ cup mozzarella cheese, shredded
- 1 teaspoon coconut flour
- ¾ teaspoon baking powder
- ¾ teaspoon pumpkin pie spice
- 2 teaspoons pureed pumpkin
- 4 teaspoons heavy whipping cream
- ½ teaspoon vanilla
- Pinch salt
- 2 teaspoons maple syrup (sugar-free)

Method:

1. Turn your waffle maker on.
2. Mix all the ingredients except maple syrup in a large bowl.
3. Pour half of the batter into the waffle maker.
4. Close and cook for 4 minutes.
5. Transfer to a plate to cool for 2 minutes.
6. Repeat the steps with the remaining mixture.
7. Drizzle the maple syrup on top of the chaffles before serving.

Nutritional Value:

- Calories 201
- Total Fat 15 g
- Saturated Fat 8 g
- Cholesterol 200 mg
- Sodium 249 mg
- Potassium 271 mg
- Total Carbohydrate 4 g
- Dietary Fiber 1 g
- Protein 12 g
- Total Sugars 1 g

Choco Waffle with Cream Cheese

Preparation Time: 5 minutes

Cooking Time: 8 minutes

Servings: 2

Ingredients:

Choco Chaffle

- 2 tablespoons cocoa powder
- 1 tablespoon almond flour
- ¼ teaspoon baking powder
- 2 tablespoons sweetener
- 1 egg, beaten
- ½ teaspoon vanilla extract
- 1 tablespoon heavy whipping cream

Frosting

- 2 tablespoons cream cheese
- 2 teaspoons confectioner's sugar (swerve)
- 1/8 teaspoon vanilla extract
- 1 teaspoon heavy cream

Method:

1. Combine all the choco chaffle ingredients in a large bowl, adding the wet ingredients last.
2. Mix well.
3. Plug in your waffle maker.
4. Pour half of the mixture into the device.
5. Close and cook for 4 minutes.
6. Cook the other waffle.

7. While waiting, make your frosting by adding cream cheese to a heat proof bowl.
8. Place in the microwave.
9. Microwave for 8 seconds.
10. Use a mixer to blend the cream cheese with the rest of the frosting ingredients.

11. Process until fluffy.

12. Spread the frosting on top of the chaffle.

13. Put another chaffle on top.

14. Pipe the rest of the frosting on top of the chaffle.

15. **Slice and serve.**

Nutritional Value:

- Calories 151
- Total Fat 13 g
- Saturated Fat 6 g
- Cholesterol 111 mg
- Sodium 83 mg
- Potassium 190 mg
- Total Carbohydrate 5 g
- Dietary Fiber 2 g
- Protein 6 g
- Total Sugars 1 g

Bacon, Olives & Cheddar Chaffle

Preparation Time: 5 minutes

Cooking Time: 8 minutes

Servings: 2

Ingredients:

- 1 egg
- ½ cup cheddar cheese, shredded
- 1 tablespoon black olives, chopped
- 1 tablespoon bacon bits

Method:

1. Plug in your waffle maker.
2. In a bowl, beat the egg and stir in the cheese.
3. Add the black olives and bacon bits.
4. Mix well.
5. Add half of the mixture into the waffle maker.
6. Cover and cook for 4 minutes.
7. Open and transfer to a plate.
8. Let cool for 2 minutes.
9. Cook the other chaffle using the remaining batter.

Nutritional Value:

- Calories 202
- Total Fat 16g
- Saturated Fat 8g
- Cholesterol 122mg
- Sodium 462mg
- Potassium 111mg
- Total Carbohydrate 0.9g
- Dietary Fiber 0.1g
- Protein 13.4g
- Total Sugars 0.3g

Sausage & Egg Chaffle Sandwich

Preparation Time: 5 minutes

Cooking Time: 10 minutes

Serving: 1

Ingredients:

- 2 basics cooked chaffles
- 1 tablespoon olive oil
- 1 sausage, sliced into rounds
- 1 egg

Method:

1. Pour olive oil into your pan over medium heat.
2. Put it over medium heat.
3. Add the sausage and cook until brown on both sides.
4. Put the sausage rounds on top of one chaffle.
5. Cook the egg in the same pan without mixing.
6. Place on top of the sausage rounds.
7. Top with another chaffle.

Nutritional Value:

- Calories 332
- Total Fat 21.6g
- Saturated Fat 4.4g
- Cholesterol 139mg
- Potassium 168mg
- Sodium 463mg
- Total Carbohydrate 24.9g
- Dietary Fiber 0g
- Protein 10g
- Total Sugars 0.2g

Swiss Bacon Chaffle

Preparation Time: 5 minutes

Cooking Time: 8 minutes

Servings: 2

Ingredients:

- 1 egg
- ½ cup Swiss cheese
- 2 tablespoons cooked crumbled bacon

Method:

1. Preheat your waffle maker.
2. Beat the egg in a bowl.
3. Stir in the cheese and bacon.
4. Pour half of the mixture into the device.
5. Close and cook for 4 minutes.
6. Cook the second chaffle using the same steps.

Nutritional Value:

- Calories 237
- Total Fat 17.6g
- Saturated Fat 8.1g
- Cholesterol 128mg
- Sodium 522mg
- Total Carbohydrate 1.9g
- Dietary Fiber 0g
- Total Sugars 0.5g
- Protein 17.1g
- Potassium 158mg

SHOPPING LIST

Pepper

Salt

Yellow onion

Eggs

Cauliflower

Mixed berries

Vanilla extract

Almond extract

Sweetener

Cream cheese

Cottage cheese

Cheddar cheese

Sugar-free barbecue sauce

Bacon

Ground beef

Parmesan cheese, grated

Almond flour

Onion powder

Garlic powder

Cauliflower crumbles

Eggs

Coconut

Pumpkin seeds

Blueberries

Butter

Dried oregano

Mozzarella

Black olives

Turkey pepperoni

Grape tomatoes

Olive oil

Cinnamon

Herbed goat cheese

Ground pork

Ground beef

Water

Whiskey

Bacon grease

Apple cider vinegar

Mayonnaise

Green onions

Red cabbage

Toothpicks

Alfalfa sprouts

Coriander

Honey

Tamari Soy Sauce

Fish Sauce

Honey

Chile garlic sauce

Fat coconut milk

Peanut butter

Swiss cheese

Mayonnaise

Dijon mustard

Sauerkraut

Corned beef

Dijon mustard

Dry thyme

Spinach

Carrots

Mushrooms

Pork

Onion

Sesame seeds

Lemon juice

Onion

Olive Oil

Parsley

chicken

beef

pork

shrimp

Water

Flaxseeds

Coconut Oil

Baking Powder

Carrot

Avocado

Lemon juice

Ginger

Strawberries

Stevia

Coconut flakes

Paprika

Blueberries

Banana

Almond milk

Tomatoes

Broccoli

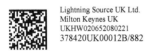

Lightning Source UK Ltd.
Milton Keynes UK
UKHW020652080221
378420UK00012B/882